AF426332

PRIORITIZE

SELF-CARE

GUIDE & WORKBOOK

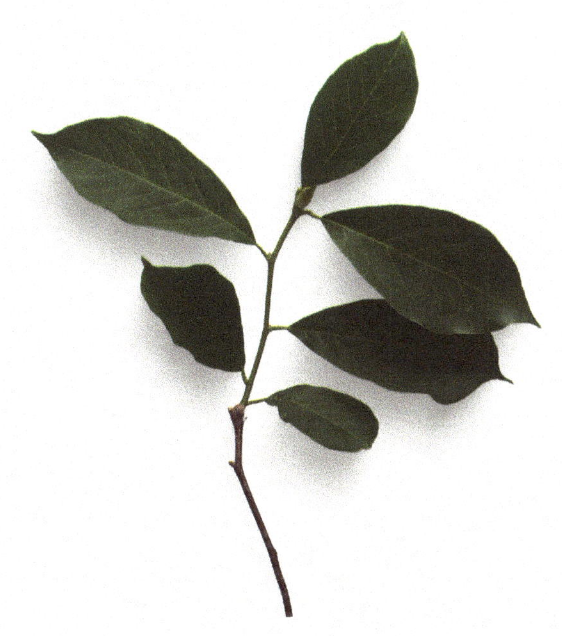

ISBN: 979-8-9865891-1-4
©2022 VIKKI JONES
VMH PUBLISHING®
WWW.VMHPUBLISHING.NET

Welcome!

What is self-care?

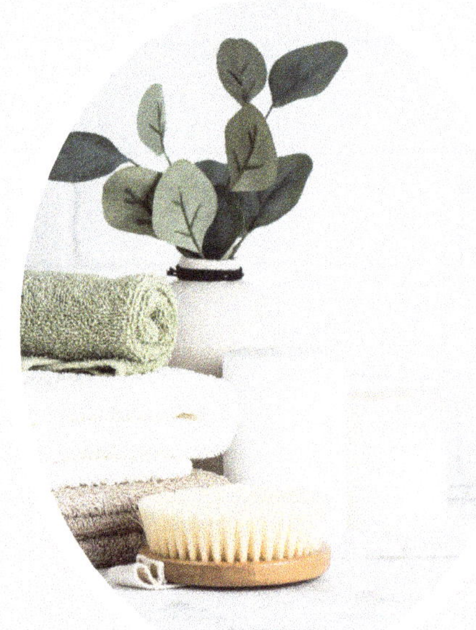

The simplest definition is that self-care is any activity which helps you to enhance your well-being and maintain your health - both physical and mental. This means self-care can be anything from eating nourishing food or getting enough sleep, to setting aside time for a creative or spiritual endeavor.

Practicing good self-care can help you to manage your moods and feel your best, with research showing that prioritizing self-care can help with managing emotions as well as increase overall physical wellness.

Taking care of yourself can make you feel more empowered, more secure, and more content with your everyday life. Even choices that seem difficult, such as setting tough boundaries or asking your family members to help you out around the house, can have long-term benefits that help you feel loved and ultimately strengthen your connections to those in your life.

Self-care is more of a lifestyle change that allows you to make time for your health in order to ensure your general well-being now and in the future. If you do embrace the proper self-care strategies, you will be able to enjoy the benefits, such as improved physical and mental health, and improved connections. 'Prioritize Self-Care Guide and Workbook' will assist with adjusting your lifestyle.

THE 7 PILLARS
of Self-Care

MENTAL

Mental self-care is about cultivating a healthy mindset through mindfulness and curiosity.

EMOTIONAL

Emotional self-care involves taking care of your heart with healthy coping strategies.

PHYSICAL

Physical self-care involves taking care of your body with exercise, nutrition and proper sleep.

ENVIRONMENTAL

Environmental self-care involves taking care of the spaces and places around you.

INSPIRATIONAL

Inspirational self-care involves activities or practices that give a sense of meaning to your life.

RECREATIONAL

Recreational self-care involves making time for hobbies, fun activities and new experiences.

SOCIAL

Social self-care involves building relationships with regular connection and healthy boundaries.

SELF-CARE IDEAS
for Yourself

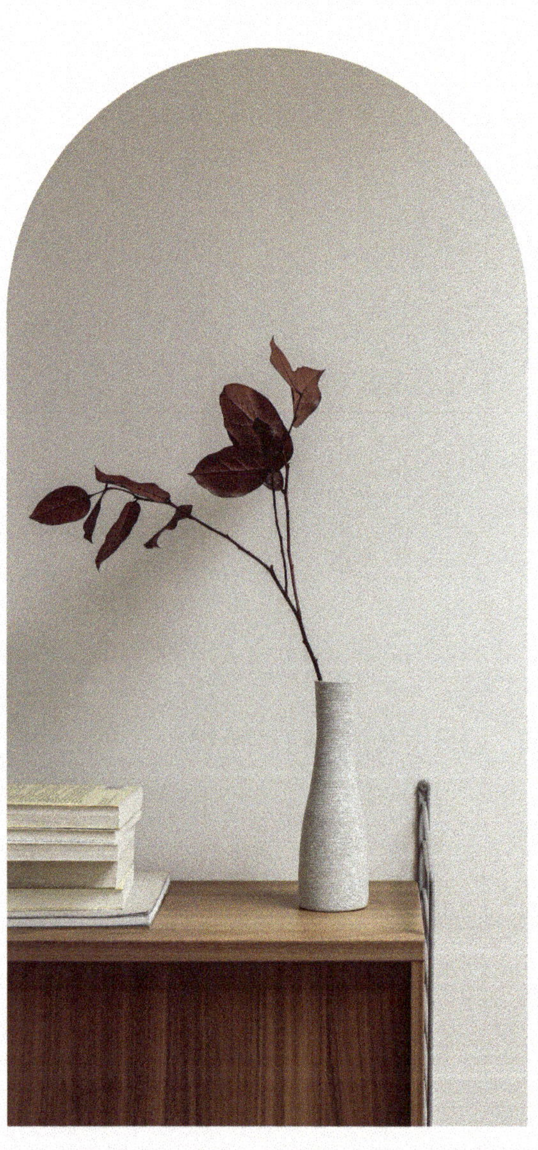

PHYSICAL

- Exercises
- Do yoga
- Go for a walk
- Get quality sleep
- Drink enough water
- Take a bubble bath

MENTAL

- Get a new experiences
- Avoid toxic people
- Explore your creativity
- Meditate
- Read a book
- Watch a movie

EMOTIONAL

- Journal
- Say positive things
- Learn to say no
- Practice gratitude
- Practice forgiveness
- Celebrate your wins

SOCIAL

- Give social media a break
- Join support group /Participate in an event
- Meet new people / Catch up with friends

INSPIRATION

- Meditate
- Help someone
- Self-reflect
- Observe quiet time
- Read inspirational books
- Spend time with nature

SELF-CARE
Assessment

Using the scale below, rate the following areas in terms of frequency.

1 = Poor 2 = Moderate 3 = Good

	1	2	3
PHYSICAL SELF-CARE			
MENTAL SELF-CARE			
EMOTIONAL SELF-CARE			
SOCIAL SELF-CARE			
INSPIRATIONAL SELF-CARE			

SELF-CARE

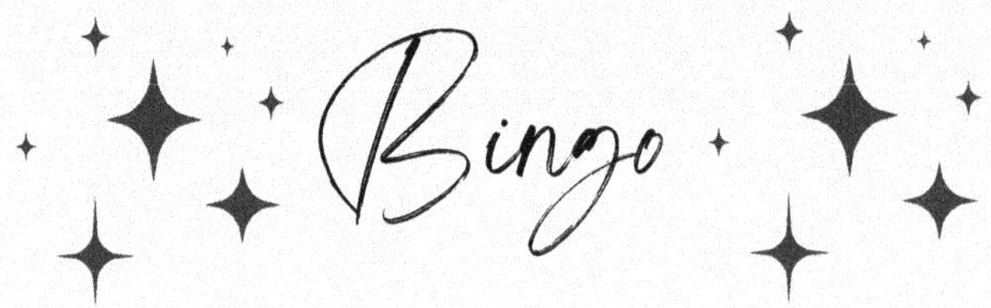

Ate a nutritious meal	Went for a walk with music or a podcast	Talked to someone you loved about important stuff	Set a goal and met it	Worked on something creative
Met with a friend for lunch or dinner	Wrote in a journal	Used a positive affirmation	Met with a group of friends	Got out from comfort zone
Workout	Rested when tired instead of pushing through	Made an appointment	Ate my favorite food without feeling guilty	Enjoyed a bubble bath, face mask or hair mask
Treated something lovely to myself	Spent time outdoors with nature	Read or listened to a book	Practiced meditation	Spent time off social media
Sang and danced to a happy song	Called a family member for a chat	Took a break and did yoga	Bought myself flowers or chocolate	Went to sleep early

HEALING JOURNAL

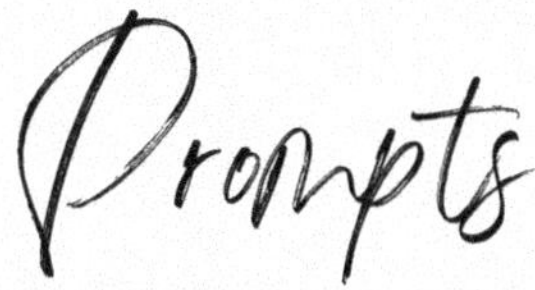

Prompts

What is weighing most on my heart right now?

What are the negative thoughts that I need to release?

What is self-care for me?

When I am alone, how do I feel?

When I am with others, how do I feel?

HEALING JOURNAL

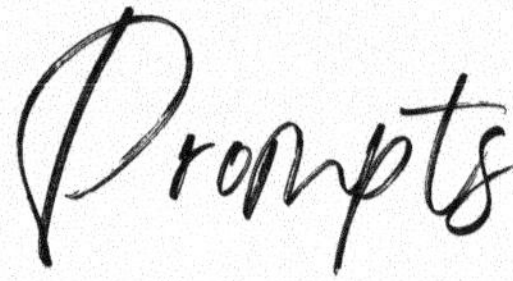

What are some habits I need to break?

What are some habits I want to start?

What is one thing I can do that will make me excited to wake up in the morning?

What do I need to forgive myself for?

Who do I need to forgive and why?

HEALING JOURNAL

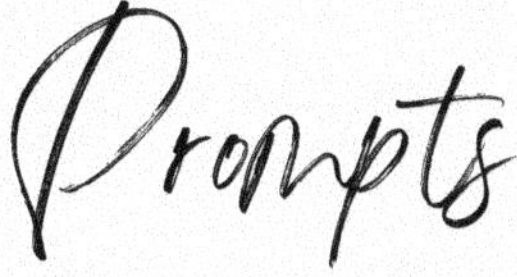

What does an exceptional day look like to me?

How can I make that a reality?

What does success look like to me?

How can I compliment my passions into my daily routine?

What is one self-care ritual I want to bring into each day?

JOURNAL PROMPTS

Daily Self-Reflection

Currently, what are my three biggest goals?

What did I do today to be one step closer to achieving them?

What is currently not helping me and needs to be removed from my to-do list?

Am I living in a way that reflects the person I want to be?

How I can make tomorrow better?

TIPS FOR HAVING A

Low-Stress Life

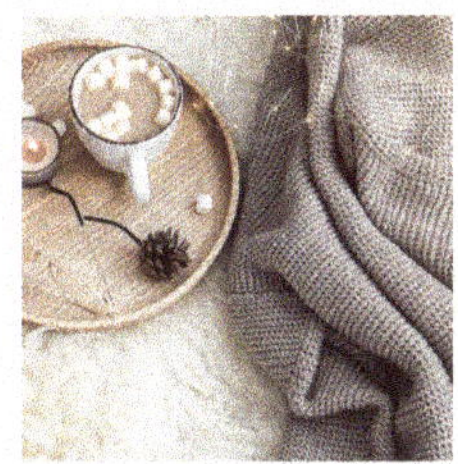

Simplify your time, your stuff and social media.

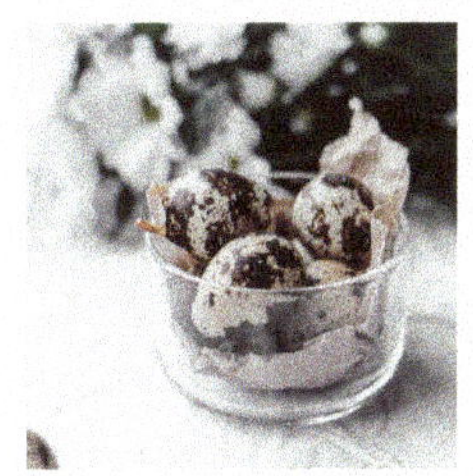

Live in the moment.

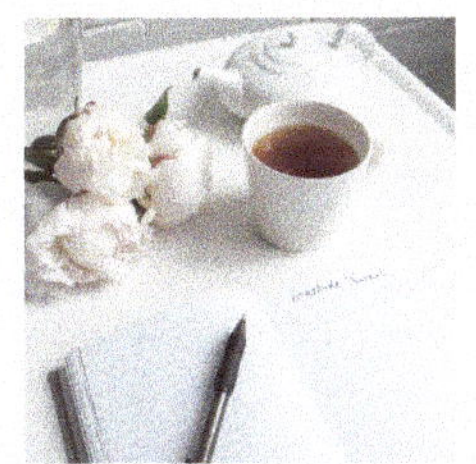

Practice gratitude.

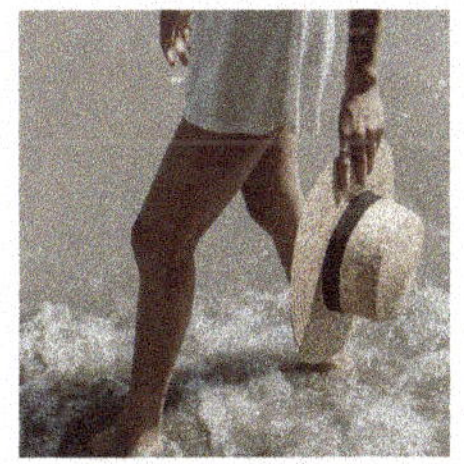

Practice getting comfortable with saying 'NO'.

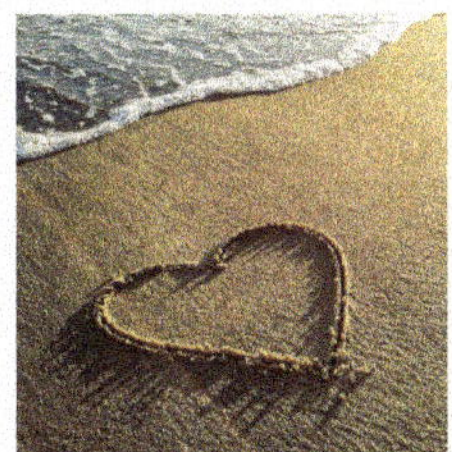

Don't worry about others, and what they think of you.

QUESTIONS TO ASK
When Faced with a Challenge

1. Is this something I should take seriously and try to make right? Is it something that is worth working on, and investing more energy on?

2. How much is my fault? Is it something I can change further down the road?

3. How much is outside of my control? Will anything I do really alter the situation or make a lasting difference?

4. Have I done everything I possibly can? Have I tried and exhausted all possible options?

QUESTIONS TO ASK
When Things Happen

5. Is it something I should put behind me, and decide to
walk away from?

6. Who else has gone through a similar experience, or had this happen to
them? Who I can talk with and give me valuable help and advice?

7. How I can build myself up again so I have the needed strength
to go forward in my life?

8. How can I learn from this experience?

HOW TO SET
Healthy Boundaries

1

LISTEN TO YOURSELF

Begin by listening to yourself. What's important to you? What are your needs? Are you feeling any resentment, anger or discomfort? These feelings are a sign of poor boundaries.

2

LEARN TO SAY NO

Give yourself permission to say 'NO'. It's absolutely okay to say no! You don't need to explain, debate or defend yourself.

3

ALLOW ROOM FOR FLEXIBILTY

Know that boundaries can be flexible. It's a balance. Too rigid, you risk isolation. Too soft, you risk exploitation. It comes back to applying Step 1 and knowing the situation before you. This is a progress towards healthy living.

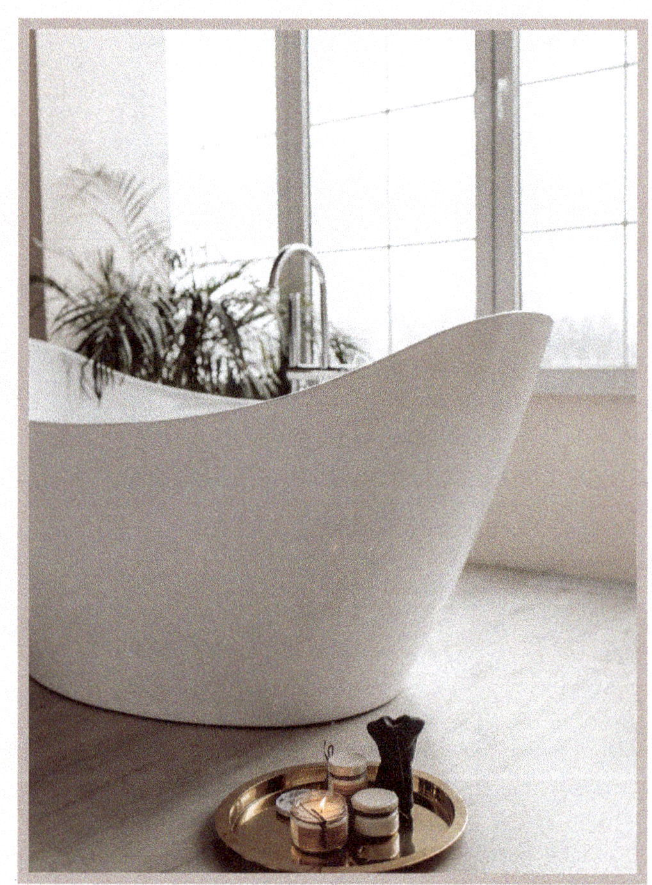

HELPFUL WAYS TO
Communicate Boundaries

- I might have to leave early.

  ⋯⋯⋯➤ I can only stay for an hour.

- I'll try to be there.

  ⋯⋯⋯➤ I won't be able to attend. Sorry.

- Okay, this is the last shot though.

  ⋯⋯⋯➤ No, thanks. I've had enough to drink.

- Yeah, I gained a few pounds. I need to lose them. I know.

  ⋯⋯⋯➤ It is not okay that you comment on my weight. I'd like you to stop .

- It's late. But sure, let's hangout.

  ⋯⋯⋯➤ It's too late now. How about another day instead?

- Oh interesting. I didn't notice that about her.

  ⋯⋯⋯➤ It is not okay with me that you gossip about my friend.

- I've got a lot of my plate. But sure, I'll do it.

  ⋯⋯⋯➤ Given my current workload. I won't be able to help you right now.

HEALTHY BOUNDARIES
Worksheet

Objectives: To help identify healthy and unhealthy boundaries in relationships and work on them.

Instructions: In the table given below, write down some of the healthy boundaries in your relationship and think of ways in which you can improve them further. In the next table, recall and write down the unhealthy boundaries of your relationship. Mention the ways in which you can replace them with healthy boundaries.

Healthy Boundaries in My Relationship	Ways to Improve Them

Healthy Boundaries in My Relationship	Ways to Replace Them with Healthy Ones

VISION BOARD
Guide

Vision boards can be used for long term goals., for the year, for the quarter of month. Decide if yours will be broad or focused on personal goals, family goals, career goals. Themed boards can be great for life events such as a wedding day or moving into a new home.

PROMPTS

1. What do you want to accomplish? Write down 5 or more goals and be specific. (*relationships, career, finances, travel, personal growth, health and etc*)

2. Look for a visual representation of each goal you listed and add these to your board. Try to choose images that you feel excited about looking at.

3. What inspires you? What is your motivation for this goal? Find visual representations of these and add them to your board. (*Your motivations are just as an important as the goal itself. Let them be true to your heart*)

4. Think of your board as a touch-point for resetting your mind. Is there a mantra or quote that you need to see or read? Choose one or more that will inspire, reassure or put you in the right frame of mind for this part of your journey.

5. What sensory elements will you experience in your goal? Pull in visual representations that compliment the setting. (*Ex. If you are relocating from New York to near the ocean in Florida the trees will be different, the scents will be different, the sounds of a bird. These are textural compliments that will add to your vision board experience.*)

6. Identify the feelings you will feel at the moment of realization or accomplishment of your goal. Either write or add visual representations of these on your board.

VISION BOARD
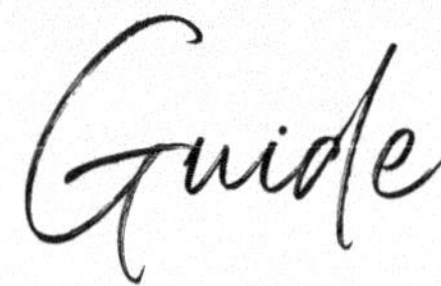
Guide

ENVISION

1 . Look at your board and soak everything in. If doubts appear, thank them for their appearance and show them out. They are not needed in this space you've created. It's your sanctuary and reprieve. Counter any negative thoughts with positive ones.

2 . Close your eyes and walk into your board. What do you see? Hear? Smell? Feel? Taste? How are you feeling there? Are you with yourself or someone else? Get detailed in the joy of the moment.

3 . Replay your vision in the morning, or before bed, when you have a quiet moment to sit or anytime you feel you need to reset your mind space. Add to it as you feel moved to.

NOTE :

Don't feel as though you need to have your entire board figured out in one sitting. Allow yourself to think, feel, breath, and grow. You may even consider intentionally leaving blank space to come back and add to your board as inspirations and ideas arise over time.

SETTING
Life Goals

For each category listed below, write down the things you are doing well, and the areas where you need improvement. Then, write a goal or two for each category.

Category	What I'm Doing Well	Where I Need Improvement	My Goals
Family			
Friends			
Work/ School			
Spiritually			
Body			
Mental Health			

PRACTICAL WAYS TO FIND YOUR

Passion & Purpose

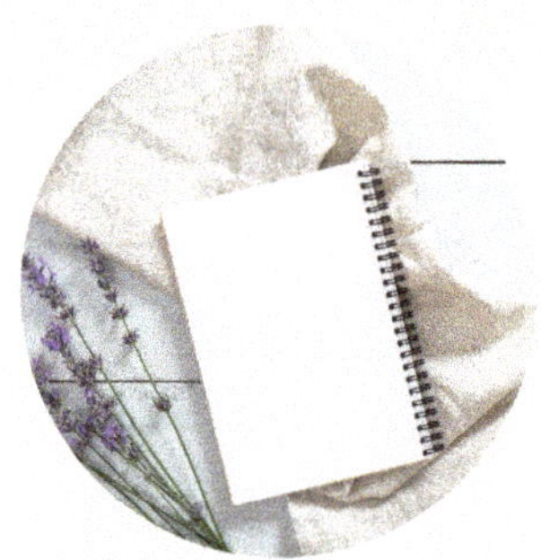

WRITE IT DOWN

Start a journal to unlock hidden thoughts of your subconscious and explore a part of you that has been dormant for a long time. Write your daily thoughts about what made you feel good that day or even what didn't make you feel good. Write a daily gratitude list for all the things that you were thankful for that day.

FIND YOUR PASSION

What are the things that make you feel great? What action or activity gives you genuine excitement? Identifying your passion allows you to begin living your purpose because your purpose comes from the way you feel when you love what you do. Are you excited to tell people what you do?

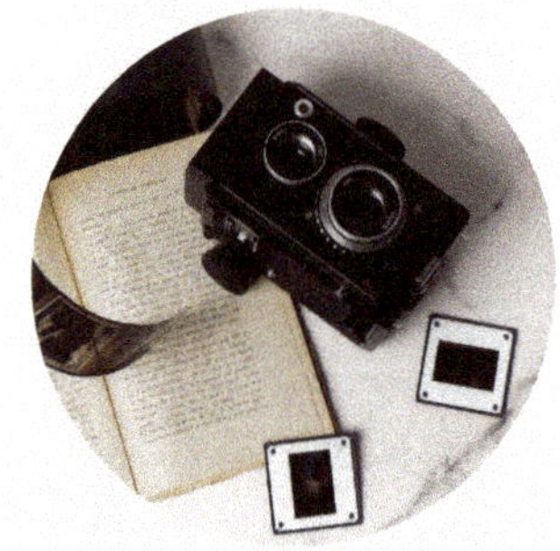

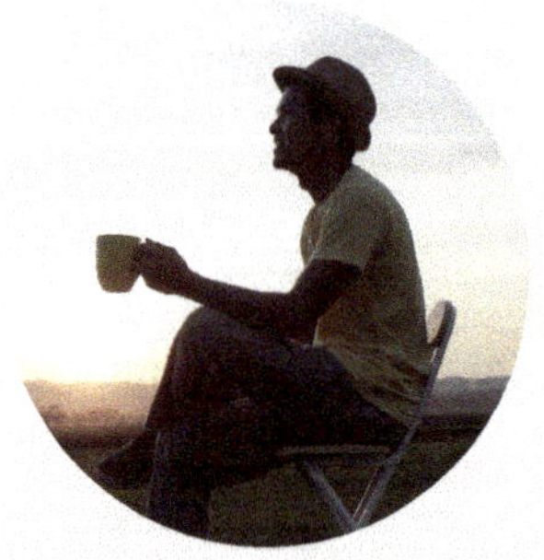

THINK ABOUT WHAT YOU WANT YOUR LIFE TO BE

What do you want your life to look like 1 year, 2 years or 5 years from now? Are you taking the necessary steps so it can look the way you want it to be? Take a look at your life right now. What changes can you make to achieve the future you're envisioning?

FIND YOUR PASSION

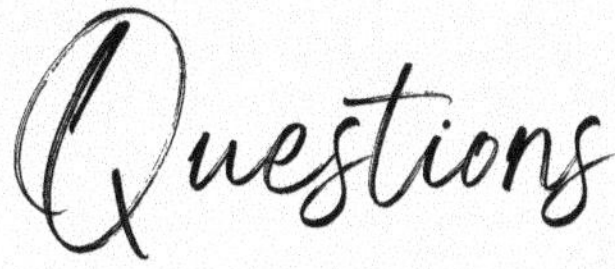

1. What was your favorite thing to do growing up?

2. When you were a child, what did you dream of doing when you grew up?

3. What is your favorite topic to talk about?

4. What do you like doing so much that you lose track of time?

FIND YOUR PASSION

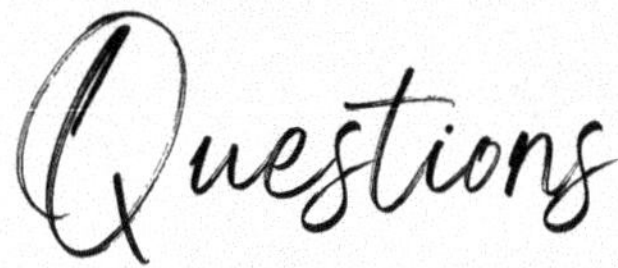

5. Whose life do you envy the most and why?

6. If you had 5 minutes and the whole world was forced to listen, what would you say?

7. What would you do with your life if you had no fear?

8. What would you do with your life if money wasn't an issue?

RELEASE & LET GO

Affirmations

I let go of what no longer serves me.

I release all limiting beliefs.

I release self-doubt.

I let go of fear.

I release attachment to outcome.

I release toxic friendships.

I let go of relationships that no longer serve my highest good.

I let go of worry.

I release lack and know that the world is abundant.

I let go of negativity.

I release all that is not in alignment with my life path.

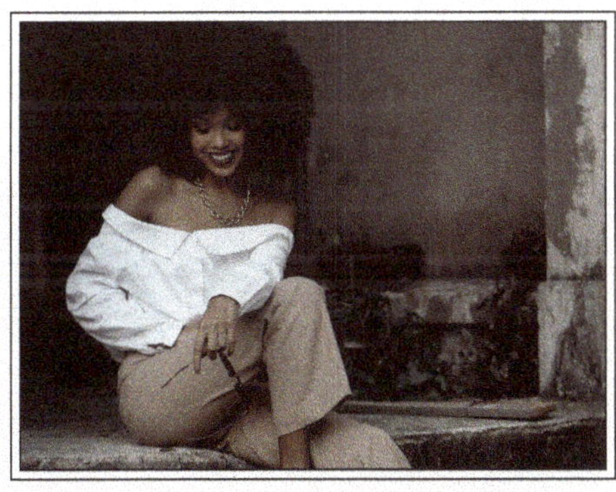

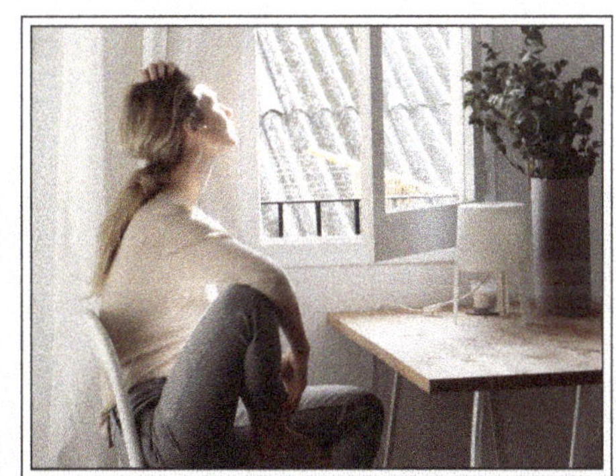

A BETTER YOU

Reminder

1. A better you is good for everyone, including you.

2. Discover something that is made just for you.

3. You deserve the time you need to be still.

4. Take your time every day to relax and renew yourself.

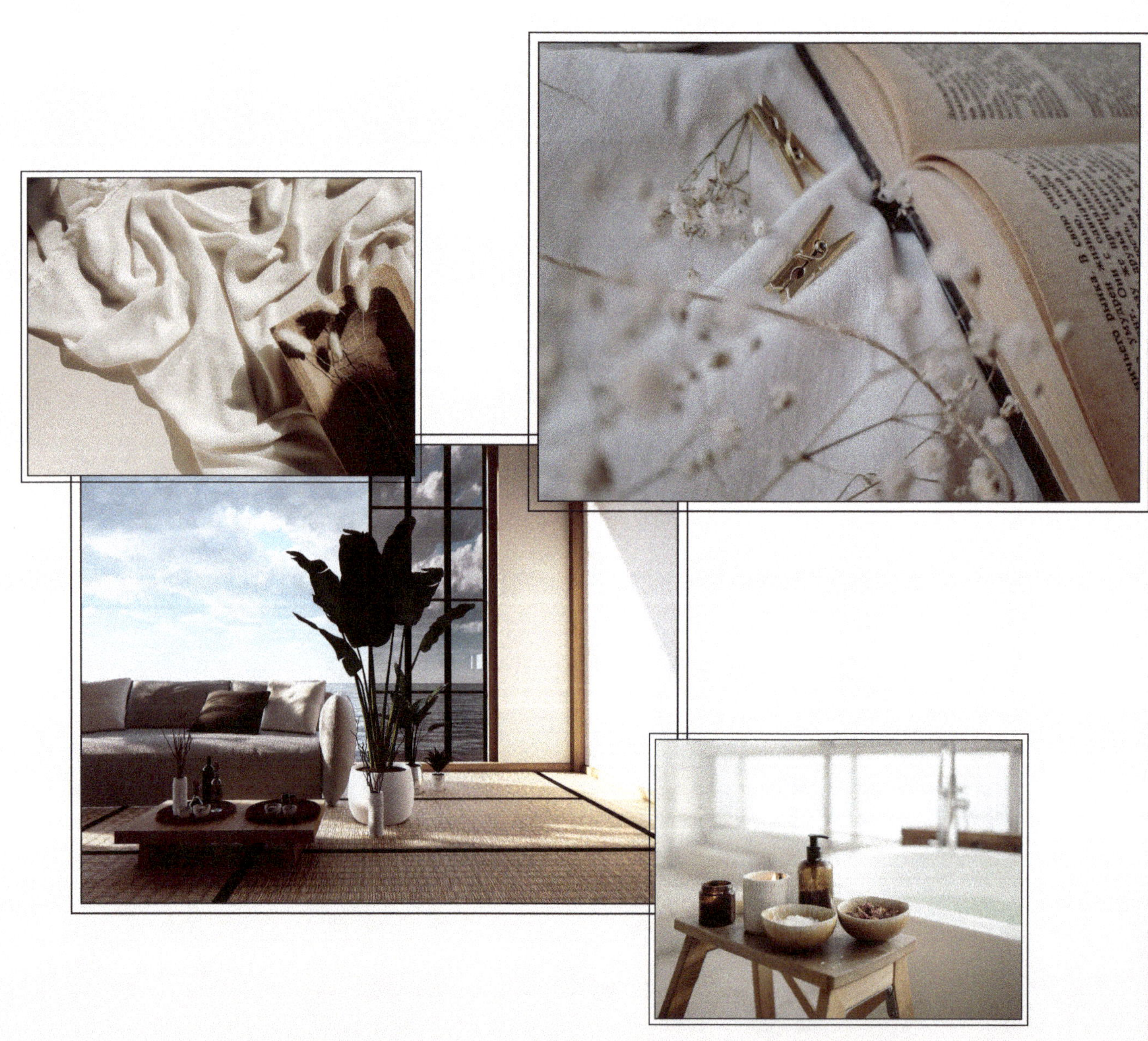

www.ingramcontent.com/pod-product-compliance
Lightning Source LLC
Chambersburg PA
CBHW041915130726
48007CB00015B/193